BLACK
CUMIN

BLACK CUMIN

*The Magical Egyptian Herb
for Allergies, Asthma,
and Immune Disorders*

PETER SCHLEICHER, M.D.

and

MOHAMED SALEH, M.D.

Translated by Nick Win Myint

HEALING ARTS PRESS
ROCHESTER, VERMONT

Healing Arts Press
One Park Street
Rochester, Vermont 05767
www.InnerTraditions.com

Healing Arts Press is a division of Inner Traditions International

First U.S. edition published in 2000 by Inner Traditions
Originally published in Germany under the title *Natürlich heilen mit Schwarzkümmel* by Südwest Verlag in der Verlagshouse Goethestrasse GmbH & Co. KG, 1998
Copyright 1998 by Südwest Verlag in der Verlagshouse Goethestrasse GmbH & Co. KG
English translation copyright 2000 by Inner Traditions International
Photographs copyright 1998 by Rolf Hayo

Note to the reader: This book is intended as an informational guide. The remedies, approaches, and techniques described herein are meant to supplement, and not to be a substitute for, professional medical care or treatment. They should not be used to treat a serious ailment without prior consultation with a qualified health care professional.

Library of Congress Cataloging-in-Publication Data

Schleicher, Peter.
  [Natürlich heilen mit Schwarzkümmel. English]
  Black cumin : the magical Egyptian herb for allergies, asthma, and immune disorders / Peter Schleicher, and Mohamed Saleh.
      p. cm.
  ISBN 978-0-89281-843-3
  1. Black cumin—Therapeutic use. I. Saleh, Mohamed, M.D. II. Title.
  RM666.B57 S3713 2000
  615'.32334—dc21

                                                99-056015

Printed and bound in the United States

10 9

Text design and layout by Priscilla Baker
This book was typeset in Stempel Schneidler and Stone Sans

Contents

ONE

Many Ailments— One Cure

UPON READING THE LONG LIST of ailments for which black cumin in its various forms (oil, seeds, capsules) is supposed to provide relief, many people react with disbelief. But black cumin's healing powers are completely real, and they do not seem so impossible once one understands that they all stem from one source—the plant's ability to stabilize and strengthen the body's immune system. Calling black cumin a magical cure would certainly be an exaggeration, but it is almost impossible to exaggerate its effectiveness.

Black cumin, also known as the "blessed seed" and "love in a mist," is an herb whose healing characteristics have been held in high regard in the Middle East for more than three thousand years. The herb was traditionally used to treat respiratory illnesses, stomach and intestinal ailments, and circulatory and immune system dysfunction, and as a tonic for general well-being. In the Bible black cumin is called "fitch," and the Prophet Mohammad stated in his Hadith that black cumin oil cures every illness except death.

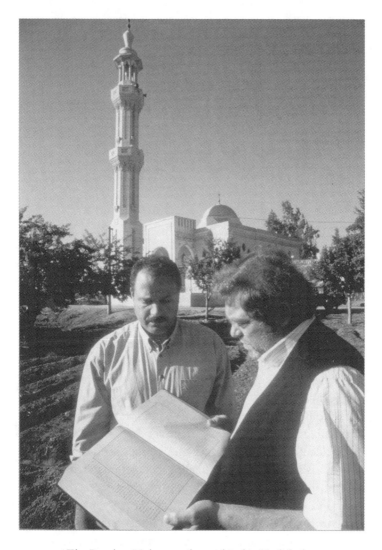

The Prophet Mohammad stated in his Hadith that black cumin oil cures every illness except death.

Black cumin was once valued highly as a healing plant and a spice in Europe as well, but it was slowly forgotten and by the eighteenth century was found in gardens for decorative purposes only. However, black cumin is experiencing a revival in the West, and researchers in Europe and the United States are now proving scientifically what people in the Middle East have always known.

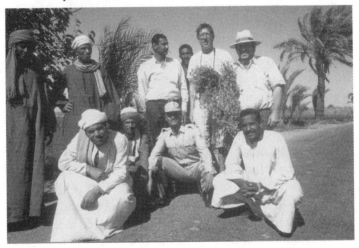

Dr. Peter Schleicher and the expedition team.

WEAKENED IMMUNE SYSTEMS— A MODERN DISEASE

Each day our body must fight off a multitude of microorganisms and pathogens, especially bacteria, viruses, and fungi. Normally we do not notice this because we have an efficiently functioning defense mechanism—our immune system. A healthy immune system reacts to attacks from the outside, fights harmful intruders, and eliminates them as quickly as possible. Only when the defense mechanism of our body can no longer function properly do the pathogens have a chance. Once they have found a basis for attack, the risk of infections and other diseases increases substantially.

Constant stress and severe psychological strains, poisons in our environment, lack of sleep or physical activity, and an unbalanced diet can all lead to a weakened immune system. Because these conditions are all but guaranteed in modern society, more and more people in the industrialized world suffer from this. The result is an increased susceptibility to colds, skin and breathing problems, overgrowth of fungi, and allergies, as well as disturbances of the digestive system, chronic exhaustion, and migraines. A causal link even exists between cancer and certain immune disturbances.

There are several ways of strengthening the immune system and preventing these diseases. Chemical preparations often have undesirable side effects and only suppress the symptoms of an illness without curing it. That is why today, more than ever, the methods of conventional medicine are being questioned. More and more people place their trust in natural methods of healing that work holistically to heal the whole person. In this book you will see how black cumin stabilizes and rebuilds your body's defense mechanism in a gentle and natural manner, without the side effects of other methods of treatment. Furthermore, you will learn how it can be used to treat the most common ailments in a way that brings permanent relief.

BLACK CUMIN—THE BASICS

The use of black cumin as a spice and healing plant can be traced back to ancient Egypt. There, it was a vital ingredient in many dishes. The personal doctors of the pharaohs always had a bowl of black cumin seeds handy, to use as a digestive aid after extensive dinners and as an effective medicine for colds, headaches, toothaches, and infections. In the grave of the pharaoh Tutankhamun archaeologists found a bottle of this ancient medicine—in preparation for life after death.

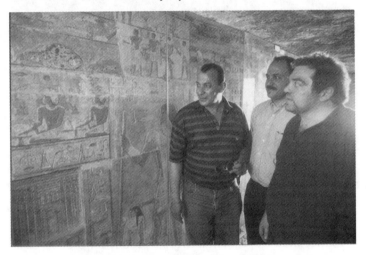

*The use of black cumin as a spice and healing plant
can be traced back to ancient Egypt.*

Black cumin (*Nigella sativa*) today is cultivated in North Africa, Asia, and southeastern Europe. The most important producers of it are Egypt, India, Pakistan, Iran, Iraq, and Turkey. The hot, dry climate and sandy soil of these countries offer ideal growing conditions for the plant, which has graceful bluish white blossoms and exotic-looking seedpods. Egyptian black cumin, the best choice for healing purposes, is cultivated in the middle of the Arab desert in extended oases. It is important that only Egyptian black cumin be used for healing purposes. Other types, such as Turkish black cumin (*Nigella damascena*), have little significance as healing herbs, and one type, *Nigella garidella,* is even poisonous.

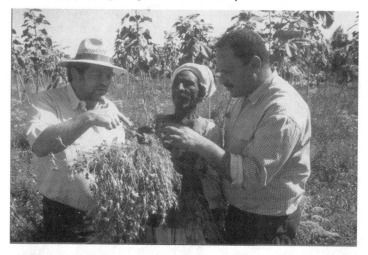

The harvest starts as soon as the plants start dying off at the bottom.

Black cumin crops intended for oil production are sowed in September. Until the plants flower the fields are watered on a regular basis. Once the seedpods have formed, watering is stopped so that the cumin can dry. The harvest starts as soon as the plants start dying off at the bottom. The seedpods at this stage are a light brown, the seeds black and hard. Plants are cut before sunrise to keep the plants from becoming wet with morning fog or dew. The cut plants are then spread out to dry in big bundles on clean sheets and are turned over at regular intervals. Finally, after being ground and bagged, the seeds are transported to the oil mill.

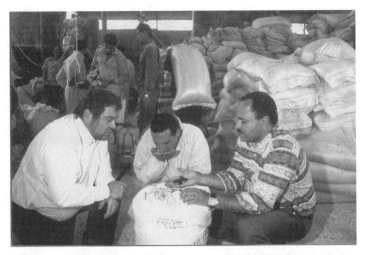

Black cumin seeds are ground and bagged
before being transported to the oil mill.

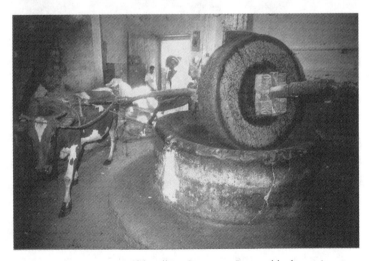

In this 350-year-old mill in Qus near Luxor, black cumin
seeds are still ground into oil the traditional way.

Black cumin oil used for therapeutic purposes must be cold-pressed. If chemically extracted at high temperatures the valuable unsaturated fatty acids are destroyed. And while the yield of cold-pressing is lower than that of chemical extraction, all valuable ingredients remain intact.

Paying Attention to Differences in Quality

Not all black cumin products are the same. The differences between the various brands are significant. Thus you should not buy any unverified black cumin oil just because it's on sale. To ensure that you are purchasing a quality product, ask the experts in the pharmacy or health store.

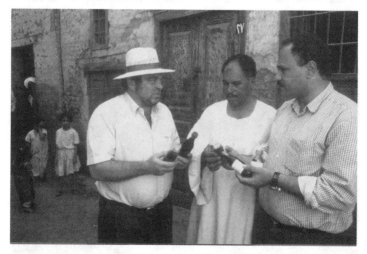

Dr. Peter Schleicher and Dr. Mohamed Saleh find that pure black cumin oil offers the most significant health benefits.

With black cumin, the medical and cosmetic effectiveness of the plant depends on the type and place of origin. Cultivation conditions—for example, quality of the soil or intensity of sunlight—also have a big influence on the qualities of the black cumin.

Proper harvesting and cold-pressing are further preconditions for the preservation of the active ingredients.

Black Cumin from Egypt

According to the most recent research, the Egyptian black cumin has the highest therapeutic effectiveness. It grows in optimal climate conditions. Egyptian black cumin not only grows with a lot of sun and on proper soil, but it also comes from a biologically controlled cultivation, and its oil is obtained using the protective cold-pressing.

The concentration of the various active ingredients of black cumin depends on the harvesting process. Different methods for the cultivation, harvest, and extraction lead to significant discrepancies. The same goes for all impurities that can occur during any of the three stages of the process. Modern methods now prevent impurities and ensure a continuous and even distribution of active ingredients in black cumin, so be sure to look for capsules that are standardized for dosage.

Standardized Dosage

Egyptian black cumin is available in different shapes and consistencies. Black cumin oil in capsules has been tested for impurities and standardized for active ingredients during the manufacturing process, which makes a precise dosage possible. When using liquid black cumin oil, which is harder to dose properly, patients should follow the recommended dosage carefully.

Botanical Characteristics

- Black cumin belongs to the family Ranunculaceae.

- The plants have a slightly hairy stem and shiny green, tripartite leaves. The flowers are at the end of the stems and are milky white, with a slightly blue or green tint at the tip.

- The slightly curved, three-edged seeds are contained in seedpods, which are surrounded by five beak-like extensions. The seeds are black and have an odor reminiscent of anise.

- Black cumin plants mature in one year and are between one and two feet tall.

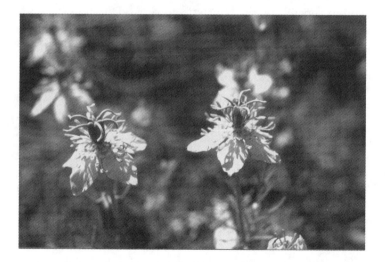

Nigella sativa *is a graceful plant with bluish white blossoms.*

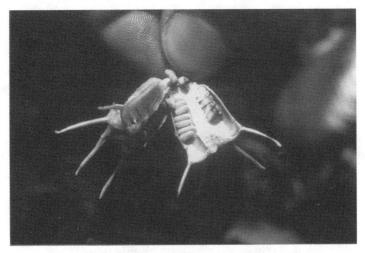

The seeds of the black cumin plant.

ACTIVE INGREDIENTS

Black cumin is an extremely complex substance containing more than one hundred ingredients, some of which have not yet been identified or studied. Its high effectiveness is due to the combination of fatty oils, volatile oils, and trace elements. It is composed of:

21 percent protein

35 percent oil (predominantly polyunsaturated fats)

38 percent carbohydrates

6 percent other ingredients

Scientists have confirmed that the active healing ingredient in black cumin is the volatile oil Nigellone. In addition to its immune-boosting properties, it is a bronchodilator and thus very effective in the treatment of asthma and whooping cough. Other important ingredients include saponin and nigellin, which give the plant its appetite-enhancing and digestion-stimulating qualities. Tannins can also be found in black cumin.

Other Ingredients in Black Cumin Oil:

alpha pinene	borneol
beta pinene	karvon
sabine	thymol
1.8-cineole	karvakrol
alpha-terpines	thynohydrochinon
p-zymes	stearin-acid
artemisiaketone	arachin-acid
sabinen hydrates	palmitin-acid
linalool	myristine-acid
beta-thujon	palmitinolein-acid
bornylazeat	behen-acid

Further active ingredients in black cumin oil include trace elements, vitamins, natural antihistamines, and natural analgesics.

Essential Fatty Acids

Black cumin is an excellent source of polyunsaturated fatty acids, especially those known as essential fatty acids, or EFAs. EFAs are vital for cell maintenance and the stabilization of cell membranes. They bring about the quick healing of wounds, contribute to smooth skin, and help metabolize cholesterol and fat in the blood. They also play an important role in the smooth functioning of the brain and the nervous system. Diets deficient in EFAs are associated with skin conditions such as acne, dandruff, and eczema, as well as more serious problems such as menstrual disorders, heart disease, and cancer.

The body uses the EFAs linoleic acid and gamma linolenic acid to produce prostaglandins—vital hormone-like substances that regulate many body processes, from T-cell production to muscle contraction and blood pressure stabilization. Prostaglandin E1 is responsible for regulating T-cell counts, thereby boosting immunity in people suffering from immunodeficiency and relieving inflammation and allergies in people suffering from overactive immune systems and high T-cell counts. Many clinical studies have shown that gamma linolenic acid also combats heart disease, reduces blood pressure, promotes weight loss, and treats diabetes, rheumatoid arthritis, and asthma. It even has been shown to kill cancer cells.

Black cumin is one of the best sources of linoleic acid and gamma linolenic acid. The only other good sources known are the oils of evening primrose, hemp seed, and borage.

A MODERN REDISCOVERY

Black cumin was rediscovered in Europe, oddly enough, because of a sick horse. A few years ago the valuable show horse Baronesse suddenly began suffering from severe asthma attacks. The horse at that time belonged to a fourteen-year-old student at the Munich Horse Academy. The owner showed the animal to several veterinarians who all suggested a cortisone-based therapy. But the owner would not consider such a therapy because of the severe side effects.

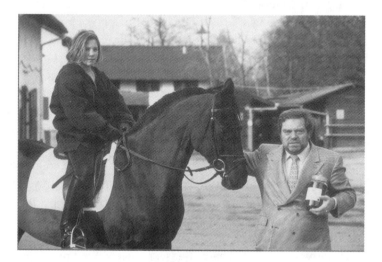

Baronesse's bout with asthma was cured by mixing black cumin seeds into her food.

Finally, the owner found a veterinarian who practiced homeopathic methods. He looked for another solution, but in spite of all his efforts he was unable to successfully treat the horse. The veterinarian contacted a doctor he knew in Egypt and asked him for homeopathic advice. The doctor said that in his country Arabian horses had been successfully cured from immune deficiencies for thousands of years with black cumin. The veterinarian mixed black cumin into the horse's food, and Baronesse quickly regained her health and soon started winning medals again.

This spectacular healing success led to the spice being examined in laboratories. Since then scientists have been analyzing exactly how black cumin works. Research is far from complete, but it is already clear today that the results of the study greatly surpass all expectations.

TWO

*Black Cumin:
The Immune
System Enhancer*

RECENT RESEARCH ON BLACK CUMIN has focused on its positive effects on the immune system. If the immune system is strengthened, numerous ailments and illnesses can be cured or alleviated. To better understand how black cumin works, a brief description of the function of the immune system is necessary.

DEFENSE OF THE BODY

Bacteria, fungi, and viruses constantly enter through the body's openings in spite of the protective mucous membranes. When this happens, the immune system is there to protect the body against these attacks from the outside.

In the lymph fluids and the blood, millions of cells that can best be thought of as specialized defense fighters circulate constantly. Some recognize enemies and sound the alarm, while others destroy the foreign invaders (antigens). These white blood cells (leukocytes) increase dramatically when an infection occurs, since it is their job to eliminate elements that cause infections. Lymphocytes, a special type of white blood cell, play the most important part in the body's defense mechanism. They are formed in the bone marrow and from there are transported to different areas of the body. In a healthy person only 5 to 15 percent of the defense cells circulate constantly in the blood and can be observed in laboratory tests. The others rest in organs and are only mobilized once antigens have been detected. There are lymphocytes in the thymus gland, the spleen, the bone marrow, the lymph gland, the tonsils, the appendix, and the lymph tissue of the intestines.

Lymphocytes are divided into B-cells and T-cells, each having separate responsibilities. B-cells form antibodies for the destruction of the intruders. Special B-cells called "memory cells" save the blueprints for these antibodies. If the same virus enters the body for a second time, the proper antibodies can thus be produced immediately—even after many years. T-cells are responsible for the actual cell-controlled self-defense: they act directly against antigens.

More than half of the T-cells in the bloodstream are helper cells. They activate the killer cells, stimulate the production of antibodies by the B-cells, and destroy those cells that have been attacked by the virus. The T-cells ensure an increased circulation of blood to the infected area, thereby bringing in reinforcements. The body temperature rises and a fever begins. Increased circulation and an increased temperature have a further advantage for the body—the heat of the fever burns the deposits of toxins that are produced in any defense response and ensures their excretion. What remains is an immune system that is now stronger than it was before. Other T-cells are suppressor cells. They make sure that there are always the proper number of helper cells circulating in the blood as needed for the various immune reactions.

The immune system can be compared to an army of attacking soldiers kept in check by defending killer cells and a controlling peacekeeping force. If a virus enters the organism, it is attacked by killer cells and destroyed. Most killer cells are destroyed in this process as well, but some remain. These active killer cells would go on to attack the cells of the body, but in a healthy organism they are prevented from doing so by the peacekeeping suppressor cells.

The immune defense works correctly only if the ratio between killer and suppressor cells is correct. If the killer cells are more numerous and are not stopped by the suppressor cells, they will attack the body's own cells. If the reverse is true, then the body's defense mechanism is too weak to fight off invaders. This results in the perfect setting for disease and chronic illness.

The consequences of too few killer cells in the blood can be:

- Susceptibility to infectious diseases

- Unsolved chronic illnesses of the digestive system, such as diarrhea

- Strange rashes or viral infections

- In the cases of those infected with HIV, the onset of AIDS

When killer cells are particularly lacking, the immune system can collapse entirely. Then a few malignant cells, which up to now have not bothered the body because they have been kept in check by the defense cells, can grow unhindered and, in the worst-case scenario, become cancer.

When the suppressor cells that in a healthy organism prevent the killer cells from taking over are too few, they are unable to stop the killer cells. The killer cells now attack the cells of the body and destroy what they are supposed to protect. This is referred to as an autoimmune reaction. The result of an excess of killer cells in the blood can be:

- Numerous forms of rheumatoid arthritis, vasculitis, spondylitis, and fibrosis of the lungs

- Leukemia

- Various forms of hepatitis, cirrhosis of the liver, and kidney problems

- Multiple sclerosis and nervous illnesses

- Epilepsy, allergies, and diabetes

ALLERGIES, ASTHMA, AND THE IMMUNE SYSTEM

One of black cumin's most promising applications is the treatment of allergies and asthma. Drugs designed to relieve the symptoms of allergies and asthma are often expensive and have troublesome side effects. Black cumin oil has been used in Asia and the Middle East for centuries as a safe, effective treatment for allergic rhinitis, asthma, bronchitis, eczema, and urticaria (hives).

Allergies and asthma usually stem from reactions to harmless substances we all encounter in daily life—various pollens, dust mites, molds, and pet dander. Seeing these substances as dangerous invaders, the immune system of the allergic person mistakenly mounts an all-out attack against them, and allergy symptoms result: sneezing, runny or stuffy nose, itchy eyes, wheezing, difficulty breathing, and, in extreme cases, collapse. In both conditions, the response of the immune system is the key.

Black cumin oil contains unsaturated fatty acids, namely linoleic acid and gamma linolenic acid, which are essential for a healthy immune system. The internal application of black cumin oil prompts a series of chemical reactions in which these unsaturated fatty acids take part. These reactions lead to the formation of arachidon-acid, a substance which in turn facilitates the synthesis of prostaglandin E1. Prostaglandin E1 suppresses the release of allergic messenger substances and harmonizes the immune system. During the course of long-term black cumin oil therapy the body's defense mechanism stops its excess activity and regains its balance. This ameliorates ailments caused by allergic hyper-reactions, such as asthma, hay fever, and eczema.

One of the most important components of black cumin oil is the active ingredient Nigellon semohiprepinon. It is an effective treatment for bronchial asthma and respiratory allergies because of its ability to expand and relax the airways. It also reduces the release of histamines into the bloodstream and thus works against allergic reactions. Another active ingredient of black cumin oil, thymohydrochinon, also acts as an antihistamine and pain reliever.

The standard diet does not supply the allergic person with the necessary amount of essential fatty acids, but long-term supplementation with black cumin oil can reduce allergic symptoms by up to 90 percent. Recent scientific research confirms that a daily intake of 500 milligrams three times a day for three to six months provides effective, low-cost therapy for those with allergies and asthma. Best of all, at this dosage black cumin oil has no side effects.

IMMUNE WEAKNESS

The increase of infections and allergies has reached serious proportions in all modern countries. More and more people suffer from cancer and AIDS. Many millions of Americans suffer from chronic states of exhaustion. All these problems have one thing in common: they are caused by disturbances in the body's immune system.

Immune deficiencies arise under severe psychological strain or continuous stress. Lack of exercise, poor diet, drugs, alcohol, cigarettes, medications, radiation, and pollutants can all play a part.

Disruptions in the immune system can become apparent in very different ways. You should consider the possibility of an immune deficiency in the case of:

- Increased susceptibility to infections

- Fungal infections

- Rashes and severe irritation, such as neurodermatitis

- Disruptions of the digestive tract, diarrhea, significant weight loss

- Frequently recurring, inexplicable aches

- Decreased performance, exhaustion

- Circulation problems, impotence

The immune-boosting power of black cumin is recommended for all these cases. If, after several weeks of black cumin therapy, you continue to suffer from exhaustion, you may have an undiscovered infection in the body that is taxing the immune system to such a degree that it can no longer function properly. Once you have localized the infection and eliminated it, you should continue with black cumin therapy for about six months so that your immune system has a chance to recover fully.

Even the Immune System Needs Practice

In the case of serious bacterial infections, antibiotics can save lives. Yet there are a number of drawbacks to using antibiotics routinely: important bacteria in the body, found mainly in the intestines, the reproductive organs, the breathing passages, and the skin, are destroyed along with the intruders. And where the natural balance of the body is disrupted, fungi and other intruders can easily settle down and spread.

By taking up the fight against harmful intruders, antibiotics cause the immune system to remain passive. While the patient may be cured from the ailment quickly, his or her immune system will become weak and therefore more vulnerable to the next infection. Moreover, the use of antibiotics often prevents the outbreak of a fever, which means that toxic substances produced during the defense processes are not excreted.

For these reasons, antibiotics should only be used when absolutely necessary. In many cases, black cumin can strengthen the body's defense mechanisms so that diseases are eliminated before antibiotics become necessary.

STUDIES CONFIRM TRADITIONAL USES

During the last forty years, more than 200 university studies and various journal articles have confirmed the traditional uses for black cumin, some of which have been in use for fourteen hundred years. Although scientists are beginning to understand more about the many ways in which black cumin works in the human body, there are still many compounds in the herb that have yet to be identified.

Scientists do know that black cumin stimulates bone marrow and immune cells and raises the interferon production, protects the body against viruses, destroys tumor cells, and inhibits infection. Research revealed that black cumin oil possesses antibiotic properties that act against a wide spectrum of gram-positive and gram-negative bacteria. In side-by-side tests with ampicillin, a common antibiotic, black cumin oil matched or exceeded the ampicillin's effectiveness in defeating gram-positive bacteria. Likewise, laboratory tests indicate that black cumin may hold promise in fighting cancer cells.

BLACK CUMIN AND CANCER

Scientists at the Cancer Immuno-Biology Laboratory of Hilton Head Island, South Carolina, are looking for a substance that kills cancerous cells without damaging the healthy tissue, as is the case during chemotherapy. The amazing results of their study are explained in the article "Study of *Nigella sativa* on Humans," the first scientific report on the cancer-fighting effects of black cumin oil. This study shows that black cumin is superior to other medicines in many regards: black cumin proved to be more effective than chemotherapy and radiation treatments—and without their serious side effects.

Ideal Substance for Cancer Prevention

The study cites several factors that make black cumin oil an ideal substance for cancer therapy and cancer prevention. The scientists found that a healthy immune system can recognize tumor cells before they endanger other cells and destroy them. Black cumin oil helps control tumors in multiple ways:

- It stimulates the production of bone marrow cells.

- It increases the production of immune cells.

- It increases the interferon production.

- Body cells are better protected against damaging influences.

- Tumor cells are destroyed.

- The number of B-cells that produce antibodies is thus increased.

Proven Successes in Cancer Therapy

The Cancer Immuno-Biology Laboratory of South Carolina ran a series of experiments in which mice were infected with tumor cells. Two thirds of the animals treated with black cumin oil were still alive thirty days after being infected. In contrast, all of the mice that did not receive black cumin treatment died in this time period.

Similarly encouraging results come from experiments with human bone marrow cells and tumor cells: a 250 percent increase of bone marrow cells and an almost 50 percent reduction in the growth of tumor cells were directly attributed to the effects of the black cumin oil therapy. The ingestion of black cumin oil is thus an effective support for every cancer therapy.

ANTIOXIDANTS

Far better than successfully treating cancer is to prevent it entirely. In addition to essential fatty acids, a number of vitamins, minerals, and trace elements are necessary for the smooth functioning of the immune system. We generally ingest these vital substances in our food. However, because of the increasing stress placed on the human organism due to pollutants and the stresses of modern lifestyles, the need for antioxidants increases. These substances protect the body cells from the onslaught of free radicals and thereby prevent the damaging oxidation processes that have been identified as a factor in heart diseases, the growth of tumor cells, early aging, and cataract formation.

The Protective Function of Antioxidants

Black cumin therapy can be especially effective in combination with a healthy diet and lifestyle that includes enough vitamins and minerals. When vitamins supplement our dietary antioxidant intake, the following advantages occur:

- They support the immune system.

- They keep the metabolism up.

- They destroy free radicals and provide protection from cancer and other diseases.

- They serve the emulation of the black cumin oil and thereby quicken its effectiveness.

- They protect the oil from oxidizing and thus from undesired changes.

- They prevent burping caused by pure black cumin oil.

Antioxidants and the Immune System

The following antioxidants are of special importance for the immune system. Adequate intake ensures that the immune system can function at peak levels, although excessive doses of any vitamin can be detrimental to the body. A full discussion of antioxidants and their functions is beyond the scope of this book, and the following list only touches on the main benefits. Because the appropriate amounts of the right supplements must be determined on an individual basis, anyone planning a supplement regimen should consult with a naturopathic physician or other qualified health care practitioner.

Beta-carotene

Beta-carotene is also known as provitamin A because the body can convert it into vitamin A as necessary. Beta-carotene promotes smooth skin and strong, shiny hair, sharpens the eyesight, and protects mucous membranes and cells. It also strengthens the immune system. The importance of vitamin A for cancer prevention has been established. Studies also show that the addition of vitamin A can bring cancerous cells back to their normal state.

Biotin

Biotin stabilizes the blood sugar level, helps relieve depression, and regulates the metabolism of fat, protein, and carbohydrates. It is also essential for healthy hair, skin, and nails.

Folic Acid

Folic acid is necessary for building red blood cells, forming amino acids essential for protein metabolism, and synthesizing substances needed for RNA and DNA. This vitamin is important for nourishing the nerves and brain, skin, hair, and bones, and mucous membranes.

Magnesium

Magnesium plays an important role in the functioning of the heart, nerve signal transmissions, muscle activity, and enzyme activity. Magnesium is needed for the formation of bones and teeth and the production of energy. Lack of magnesium can have a negative impact on the immune system.

Selenium

Selenium assists in the body's detoxification from heavy metals, improves the structure of skin and hair, strengthens the heart and circulation, and increases concentration. It also provides immune protection. Lack of selenium increases the susceptibility to cancer as well as to allergies.

Vitamin B_1

Vitamin B_1 is the ultimate energy vitamin. It helps generate energy from carbohydrates, accelerates the healing of open wounds, eases pain, and strengthens the muscles in the heart, intestines, and skeleton. Vitamin B_1 is essential for a healthy nervous system and a deficiency can lead to depression. It also enhances memory and mental alertness.

Vitamin B_2

Our bodies store very little of this vitamin, so it must be consumed on a regular basis. Vitamin B_2 is necessary for enzymes to initiate the energy production from substances such as protein, fat, and carbohydrates. It is important for skin, hair, and nails, protects the mucous membranes, and strengthens vision. Vitamin B_2 plays an important role in the production of blood and in cellular growth. Symptoms of vitamin B_2 deficiency include chapped lips, cracks at the corners of the mouth, bloodshot eyes, and scaly or oily patches on the skin.

Vitamin B_6

This vitamin strengthens the heart, muscles, circulation, and nerves. It protects the mucous membranes, fuels protein metabolism, and enhances the immune system. Symptoms of vitamin B_6 deficiency are the same as those for vitamin B_2 deficiency. A lack of vitamin B_6 can also lead to depression and anxiety.

Vitamin C

Vitamin C plays an important role in the formation of collagen, the substance that binds the cells. It also helps the body metabolize amino acids, folic acid, iron, and fats. Vitamin C strengthens the connective tissue, accelerates healing of wounds, and promotes healthy teeth and strong bones. Among the warning signs for a lack of vitamin C is an increased susceptibility to infections. Stress—psychological and physical—depletes the body of vitamin C stores, so it's a good idea to take a supplement daily.

Vitamin E

Vitamin E's actions in the human body are even more complicated than that of most vitamins. Vitamin E is fat soluble, which means that it is stored in the body's fatty tissue, muscle, liver, adrenal and pituitary glands, heart, lungs, and reproductive organs. As an antioxidant, vitamin E joins with enzymes to protect the lungs from pollution, prevent tumor growth, and protect breast, eye, liver, and skin tissues from damage.

Zinc

Zinc fosters the growth of smooth, healthy skin and strong, soft hair. It accelerates the healing of wounds and regulates the reproductive organs. About 70 enzymes in the body contain zinc. The mechanisms of our immune system all require zinc to function properly. Symptoms of zinc deficiency include white spots on the fingernails or brittle nails, acne and other skin problems, and slow wound healing. Internally, zinc deficiency causes an increased number of killer cells and a decreased number of suppresser cells. A lack of zinc leads to a reduction of the lymphocytes and thus to an increased susceptibility to virus infections.

STRENGTHENING THE IMMUNE SYSTEM WITH BLACK CUMIN

Some people need only be caught in the rain to catch a cold, which quickly turns into a serious infection. And even after the body has fought the infection successfully, a new virus makes the rounds. The consequence: you recover only to get sick again. A chronic susceptibility to infections often has psychological roots as well: people who are under extreme stress tend to be much more susceptible to illness.

Recent scientific research confirms black cumin's antibacterial and antiviral effects. Long used as a traditional remedy for colds and viral infections, black cumin is still a best bet against illness. Chapter 3 includes remedies for fighting colds and the flu naturally. In contrast to synthetic cold and flu medications, using black cumin to overcome a cold can help strengthen the immune system so that your body is able to heal more quickly and to resist additional infections.

Black cumin, when taken as part of a lifestyle that includes a healthy diet and regular exercise, can work wonders for the immune system. For example, taking 2 capsules or 25 drops of black cumin oil 3 times a day for up to 6 months can provide a general boost to the immune system if you are feeling run down.

THREE

*Applications
from A to Z*

THE FOLLOWING CHAPTER covers in alphabetical order the conditions for which black cumin can provide relief and gives tips for self-treatment of minor ailments. For more severe health problems, you should consult a doctor for accurate diagnosis and treatment. Although it possesses remarkable healing qualities, black cumin cannot replace medical treatment.

> **Caution: Black cumin seeds have traditionally been used, in large amounts, to bring on late menses. Thus, black cumin should not be used during pregnancy.**

ACNE

Acne is one of the most common chronic skin disorders, usually affecting the face and sometimes the back, chest, and shoulders as well. It consists of various kinds of blemishes and if severe can cause permanent scarring. Acne is more common among males, with the onset usually at puberty. Males are affected by acne more often than females because male sex hormones, such as testosterone, stimulate its formation, but women often experience breakouts at certain points in the menstrual cycle or during pregnancy.

Because acne often shows up during the teenage years, those who suffer serious cases may feel deep distress and may even develop emotional problems as a result. The attempt to cover the pimples with makeup or to pick or squeeze them usually fails and leads to more severe infections.

In the most common type of acne, *acne vulgaris*, cells that line the hair follicle start producing an excess of karatin and sebum, which leads to a blockage of the canal. Once the canal is blocked, conditions are perfect for a bacterium called *Propionibacterium acnes* to overgrow and cause inflammation. When the bacterium grows out of control, pustules or pimples form on the surface of the skin. An unhealthy diet and tension may aggravate acne.

Dermatologists often recommend treatment with antibiotics, which can lead to an imbalance in intestinal flora and the development of antibiotic resistance later on. A holistic approach can resolve the condition safely.

Magic Weapon Against Skin Problems

With black cumin, skin problems can be countered early on. Usually symptoms will diminish after about two weeks of regular ingestion of black cumin. Take 1 or 2 capsules or 25 drops of black cumin oil 3 times a day. External application of black cumin cream will reduce scarring and discourage breakouts.

Eliminating all refined sugars, reducing the consumption of high-fat foods, and limiting milk consumption may also help. A number of vitamins, including vitamins A and E and zinc, may also reduce the severity of breakouts. Increasing intake of fresh foods rich in these vitamins—such as almonds, apricots, beans, beef, cantaloupe, carrots, cheese, dandelion greens, kale, oats, and olive oil—may be beneficial for the healing of the skin.

BLACK CUMIN CREAM

8 ounces (240 ml) apple cider vinegar
1 cup (227 g) finely ground black cumin seeds

Mix the apple cider vinegar with the ground black cumin seeds and let the mixture steep for 6 to 7 hours. Filter the mixture through cheesecloth and let the solution sit for a day while the sediment settles at the bottom. Carefully pour out the liquid on top. Mix the remaining sediment in a 1:1 ratio with black cumin oil. Then heat the mixture for 2 to 3 minutes and mix thoroughly. Store in a glass jar in the refrigerator.

Apply the cream several times a day to the affected skin area. The cream is most effective when it is applied before going to bed or after a facial steam bath.

D. S., a seventeen-year-old female, had severe acne on her forehead, cheeks, and chest. Standard acne creams did not reduce the incidence or severity of the breakouts. She started taking two capsules of black cumin oil three times a day, and within four weeks her skin condition began to improve. After three months, her skin was clear.

ALLERGIES AND HAY FEVER

Allergies are caused by an overreaction of the immune system to a substance that is normally harmless. The body's defense mechanism is no longer able to tell the difference between harmless and dangerous intruders and fights all foreign substances. Common forms of allergy include asthma (discussed on pages 37–40), seasonal allergic rhinitis (hay fever), and perennial allergic rhinitis, which causes symptoms year round. In severe cases, even passing contact with the allergy-causing substance (allergen) will cause an immediate reaction. The allergens that usually cause the most respiratory problems include dust mites, mold spores, pollen, and animal dander from pets.

Contact with an allergen causes the body to produce proteins called antibodies, which stimulate the release of histamine and other substances from body cells into the bloodstream and body fluids. The allergy sufferer then experiences the familiar runny or stuffy nose; sneezing; itching, burning eyes; and hives or eczema. In extreme cases, breathing difficulties, asthma attack, or anaphylactic shock can ensue.

Allergic reactions can be aggravated by:

- General weakness of the immune system
- Unhealthy diet
- Allergy to certain foods
- Damaged intestinal flora
- Slow enzyme activity
- Genetic predisposition
- Toxins or allergens in the environment
- Constant psychological stress
- Other factors

Black Cumin for Allergy Relief

Black cumin oil has proven successful in treating seasonal allergies. In numerous cases, patients who routinely experienced severe reactions to pollen each spring remained completely free of symptoms after the regular ingestion of black cumin oil. Black cumin oil provides the necessary additional amount of unsaturated fatty acids that people who suffer from allergies need to balance their overactive immune systems (see chapter 2).

If treatment with black cumin oil starts several weeks before the pollen season begins, seasonal allergy sufferers often find significant relief from symptoms. The daily dose of black cumin oil is 1 or 2 capsules 3 times a day or 20 to 25 drops 3 times a day. For best results, begin treatment in January because it will take about 2 weeks before results are apparent. Continue treatment through the summer months.

If the allergic reaction is already in progress, a black cumin inhalation will provide more immediate relief. The allergic person should continue to take black cumin internally throughout the allergy season, using black cumin tea and inhalations for additional relief as needed.

BLACK CUMIN INHALATION

1 cup (227 g) finely ground black cumin seeds
1 quart (1 l) boiling water

Put the black cumin seeds in a glass or ceramic bowl and add the boiling water. Stir briefly and allow the mixture to steep for about 5 minutes.

Wash your face and tie your hair back if it is long. Drape a large bath towel over your head to create a tent and lean over the bowl. Relax and breathe in the steam deeply.

Continue the inhalation treatment for 10 minutes. Repeat several times a day, the first time upon waking if possible. A last inhalation before going to bed ensures a quiet and restful sleep.

BLACK CUMIN TEA

1 tablespoon finely ground black cumin seeds
1 teaspoon (5 g) licorice
1 teaspoon (5 g) crushed anise seeds
1 tablespoon black or green tea leaves (decaffeinated if
    you prefer)
1 pint (50 ml) water

Mix the ground black cumin seeds with the licorice, crushed anise seeds, and black or green tea. Add the tea ingredients to a teapot or bowl. Pour a pint (50 ml) of very hot, but not quite boiling, water over the herbs and steep for 10 minutes. Sweeten with honey if desired.

Drink 1 cup of tea 3 times a day before meals for 4 to 6 weeks. The tea can also be used as an inhalation.

Caution: Large doses of licorice taken over an extended length of time may have adverse effects on anyone suffering from hypertension or kidney or liver disease. Eliminate licorice from the recipe if you have any of these conditions and consult your health care practitioner for advice. Pregnant women should avoid using licorice.

E. J., a twelve-year-old girl, was suffering from intense allergic reactions. She experienced nasal congestion, watery and itchy eyes, severe headaches, and difficulty breathing. Her doctor diagnosed her as allergic to her cat, but she was also reacting for the first time to airborne pollens during hay fever season. The girl was too sick to attend school and even mild exercise exacerbated her symptoms. Her condition only improved in closed rooms with humidifiers. Without her cat, the girl was distraught and depressed.

As part of her treatment, E. J. played with her cat for a full day, and then she was given an autologous blood injection (her own blood was drawn and reinjected). In addition, she took two capsules of black cumin oil three times a day and drank black cumin tea with a little fresh black cumin oil.

After only four days, the girl's condition had improved significantly and she was able to stop taking cortisone sprays. The autohemotherapy offered a permanent cure to her allergy to cat dander, and black cumin oil relieved the acute symptoms. E. J. continued to feel better and became active in sports. All allergic symptoms have disappeared, and she can play with her cat without a problem.

ASTHMA

Asthma is an allergic disorder characterized by a spasm of the bronchi (airway tubes in the lungs), swelling of the mucous lining of the lungs, and excessive production of a thick, clear mucus. During an asthma attack the airways become narrower and breathing becomes very difficult. The asthmatic person experiences shortness of breath, tightness in the chest, coughing, wheezing, or some combination of symptoms. Warnings that an asthma attack is occurring or may occur soon include:

- Difficulty speaking
- Blue or gray tongue or lips
- Blue fingernails
- Flared nostrils
- High pulse
- Wheezing, or, more serious, wheezing stops without other symptoms abating

Causes and Possible Consequences

Among patients up to age forty, 90 percent have asthma caused by allergies. As with seasonal and perennial allergic rhinitis, common allergens include dust mites, molds, pet dander, and various pollens. A diet high in fats and salt and low in fresh vegetables also seems to make people more vulnerable to asthma. While there is almost always an external cause for asthma, the mental or emotional state does play a role in the frequency of attacks. Constant stress and anxiety can lower the allergic threshold, triggering an attack after more moderate contact with an allergen. Panic also certainly intensifies an asthma attack.

Acute asthma attacks can be life-threatening, so it is important not to self-treat the condition. If chronic asthma is not treated effectively, it can result in permanent damage to the lungs. Fortunately, holistic treatments can be used in conjunction with potentially life-saving asthma drugs with the ultimate goal being to shore up the immune system and reduce the incidence of attacks.

Black Cumin for Asthma Relief

The essential oils in black cumin have a mucus resolving and vasodilating effect, thus providing rapid relief from acute problems. Black cumin oil relaxes the airways and reduces the release of histamines into the bloodstream. Black cumin helps heal bronchial asthma by combating the root of the problem: stabilizing the immune system (see chapter 2).

The recommended dose of black cumin oil for asthma is 2 capsules or 25 drops 3 times a day. Continue this dose for 4 to 6 months, then take a break for 2 months before starting the treatment again. Black cumin inhalations or black cumin tea, taken several times a day, will also be helpful in opening up the airways (see pages 35–36).

BLACK CUMIN SYRUP

1 small clove of garlic
2 tablespoons (30 ml) honey
1 teapoon (5 g) finely ground black cumin seeds

Crush the garlic with a garlic press or a fork and mix it with the honey and ground black cumin seeds. If desired, warm the honey in order to make the syrup more liquid.

Take 1 teaspoon of the syrup daily before breakfast and continue the treatment for about 3 weeks.

You can also use black cumin syrup to prepare a tasty and healing tea. For this, you can simply dissolve a spoonful of syrup in a cup of black or herbal tea.

You can also use black cumin syrup as the basis for an especially effective inhalation by diluting the entire mixture in 1 quart (1 l) hot water.

> **Caution: An acute asthma attack is a medical emergency and may be fatal. If you are suffering from an acute attack, consult your physician or call an emergency room immediately. If you suffer from asthma, consult your doctor before discontinuing any prescription asthma medication.**

At three years of age, L.W. developed severe hay fever with nasal symptoms and itchy, watery eyes. The onset of hay fever occurred after the boy was given antibiotics. Later that spring he suffered from additional respiratory infections and asthma and was given more antibiotics. His health continued to deteriorate as asthma attacks and infections became regular occurrences, and by the time he was five, the sick child was socially withdrawn and had trouble sleeping.

A holistic approach was necessary to restore the boy's damaged immune system to a healthy state. He was treated with black cumin oil (two capsules three times a day) and black cumin inhalations to clear the lungs. He also received autohemotherapy (a therapeutic injection of his own blood) and medication to stimulate intestinal cleansing.

After twelve days of treatment with black cumin oil, L.W.'s condition had improved significantly. Although his eyes were still irritated, his asthma had disappeared completely. After three months of therapy, the child had recovered completely from both physical and developmental problems—he now plays with friends and enjoys school. His family continues to use black cumin as a cooking oil and as a tea.

BRONCHITIS

Bronchitis is an infection of the bronchioles, the airways in the lungs, and it usually occurs in conjunction with respiratory infections. To fight the infection, the body provides the tissue of the mucous membranes with more blood. The tissue swells, making breathing more difficult. Common accompanying ailments are fever and severe coughing as well as chest and shoulder pains. If there is a high fever or severe breathing problems, a doctor must be consulted immediately.

Alleviating Annoying Coughs

Black cumin has mucus dissolving and vasodilating effects, which alleviate the symptoms of bronchitis. Take 2 capsules or 25 drops black cumin oil 3 times a day. Additionally, black cumin inhalations may relieve respiratory congestion (see pages 35, 43).

Alternatively, black cumin syrup may be taken—1 teaspoon a day before breakfast for 3 weeks—to relieve symptoms (see page 39). Black cumin tea will also help to relieve coughing (see page 36). Drink 2 to 4 cups per day.

A warm foot-bath on cold days helps prevent lung infections, and the clean air at the ocean or in the mountains has a good effect as well. You might also add "lung herbs" such as thyme or marjoram to foods when cooking.

P. W., a seventy-two-year-old male, suffered from bronchitis since the age of twenty. He was a heavy smoker with a chronic cough and frequent respiratory infections, and an X-ray revealed mild pulmonary emphysema. Tired of antibiotics and steroid inhalers, he began taking two capsules of black cumin oil three times a day. After four weeks, the chronic cough stopped, and he has had only two episodes of bronchitis in four years. He no longer needs antibiotics or inhalers.

COLDS AND FLU

The common cold and influenza (the flu) are caused by virus infections of the upper breathing passages. The pathogens are passed from person to person through sneezing, coughing, or skin contact. Generally speaking, you can get a cold or the flu at any time of the year, but during the winter the risk is especially high. The reason for this is that during the winter months the feet frequently get cold, and then the nervous system reacts by reducing blood flow to the breathing passages. The defense of the mucous membranes is reduced, and pathogens have an easier time entering the organism.

While these infections are contagious, colds are usually harmless: typical symptoms include coughing, sneezing, sore throat, hoarseness, moderate fever, headaches, and joint pains. Influenza is much more dangerous and has more pronounced symptoms accompanied by a high fever.

Strengthening the Immune System for the Cold Season

Black cumin helps the body overcome infections more quickly and ensures a speedy recovery. By strengthening the immune system black cumin also contributes to preventing complications such as ear or sinus infections or bronchitis. By harmonizing and improving the body's defense mechanism, black cumin can minimize or prevent the outbreak of an infection.

Support your immune system by taking 1 or 2 capsules or 25 drops of black cumin oil 3 times a day. If you have already been infected, take 2 capsules 3 times a day. Drink black cumin tea 3 to 4 times a day during the acute phase of the infection; when the symptoms are not present, drink 1 cup a day (see page 36). Black cumin inhalations can relieve nasal and chest congestion and soothe a cough (see below and page 35). It's also a good idea to take a vitamin C supplement (500–1,000 milligrams can be taken every 2 hours unless it causes gas or diarrhea) and to eat foods rich in vitamin C such as kiwis, oranges, grapefruits, tomatoes, and bell peppers.

INHALATION FOR INFECTIONS

1 clove of garlic
2 tablespoons (15 ml) honey
1 teaspoon (5 g) finely ground black cumin seeds
1 quart (1 l) boiling water

Crush the garlic in a bowl with a garlic press or a fork and mix with honey and ground black cumin seeds. Add the boiling water and let stand for 10 minutes.

Wash your face and tie your hair back if it is long. Drape a large bath towel over your head to create a tent and lean over the bowl. Relax and breathe in the steam deeply for 15 minutes. Repeat up to 3 times a day.

As an alternative, you may use the black cumin inhalation on page 41 to fight off an infection.

CONCENTRATION DEFICIENCY

Concentration problems are not limited to the elderly. More and more young people are having difficulty concentrating on one task for an extended period of time. Two factors are responsible for this: the physiological cause is lack of oxygen and nutrients to the brain; the psychological causes include stress, pressure, and internal conflicts that lower the ability to concentrate.

Regular black cumin use ensures that you will keep a clear head even in old age. The recommended dosage for concentration and memory is 2 capsules or 25 drops of black cumin oil 3 times a day.

You can also use black cumin like an essential oil: evaporate 4 to 8 drops of black cumin oil (in water) in an aromatherapy diffuser every day. Other essential oils that are beneficial for the mind are rosemary, basil, laurel, and peppermint.

The following internal recipe has been successful for concentration deficiencies.

BLACK CUMIN FOR MIND POWER

1 tablespoon (15 g) finely ground black cumin seeds
1 tablespoon (15 g) myrrh

Mix the ground black cumin seeds with the myrrh. Place in a dark glass and keep cool and dry.
   Take 1 teaspoon (5 g) 3 times a day with meals.

COUGH

Coughing is a vital protective reflex. It serves to expel foreign substances as quickly as possible from the breathing passages.

If during an infection pathogens collect in the lungs, the body attempts to expel them along with the cough secretions. This prevents a follow-up illness or other complications.

Smokers may experience severe coughing with heavy phlegm, especially in the mornings. Because this cough builds up over time, it is unfortunately not taken seriously enough by a lot of people.

Strengthening the Bronchial Mucous Membranes

Black cumin dissolves mucus and dilates blood vessels. This facilitates productive coughing. The herb's stabilizing influence on the immune system also facilitates healing from a cough. The recommended dosage is 2 capsules or 25 drops of black cumin oil 3 times a day. Inhaling with black cumin or taking black cumin syrup can also help (see pages 35, 39). In addition, hot black cumin tea (see page 36) acts to dissolve mucus. Try taking 1 or 2 cups as needed throughout the day.

CHRONIC FATIGUE SYNDROME

The mysterious chronic fatigue syndrome (CFS) is characterized by severe exhaustion, which may persist for months or recur periodically. While affected, patients often lack the energy to perform most of their normal daily activities, and the disease can have a serious impact on their personal and professional lives. Other symptoms include muscle and joint pain, headaches, confusion, depression, and anxiety.

The cause of CFS has not yet been determined. Various factors may be involved, including viral infection, stress, environmental toxins, vitamins or mineral deficiency, or allergies.

Conventional treatment usually consists of drugs to stimulate the immune system.

Getting New Energy with Black Cumin

Since many factors contribute to CFS, no single therapy has been proposed as of yet. One common finding in individuals who suffer from CFS is an overgrowth of *Candida albicans* in the intestinal tract (see pages 53–54). Alternative therapies focus on supporting the immune system to foster general healing. Meditation and yoga can provide relief, especially for exhaustion and lack of concentration.

The immune system can be regulated through the ingestion of 1 or 2 capsules or 20–25 drops of black cumin oil 3 times a day.

BLACK CUMIN FOR FATIGUE

2 tablespoons (30 g) black cumin seeds
1 tablespoon (15 g) royal jelly

Grind the black cumin seeds and place in a bowl. Add the royal jelly and mix well. Store the mixture in a dark glass container in a cool place (but not in the refrigerator).

Take 1 teaspoon (5 g) 2 times a day, before breakfast and lunch, for 4 weeks.

DIABETES

Diabetes is one of the leading causes of death in North America, and 12 million people suffer from the disease. *Diabetes* usually refers to *diabetes mellitus*, the most common type of the disorder, which affects the metabolism of carbo-hydrates, fats, and proteins. When the body is functioning normally, the hormone insulin enables the body to store sugar quickly. Diabetes can occur when the pancreas does not se-crete enough insulin or if the cells of the body become resis-tant to insulin. In these cases, excess sugar builds up in the blood. One of the main symptoms of diabetes is excessive urination. Other signs include greater than average thirst or hunger and weakness or loss of weight.

Diabetics may be insulin dependent (Type I diabetes) and require injections of insulin to keep the body from collapsing in shock (diabetic coma). This form of the disease often begins in childhood and must be managed carefully. How-ever, diabetes can also appear later in life and affect people with normal or average production of insulin (Type II diabe-tes). This noninsulin–dependent diabetes is a much milder form of the disease and is associated with obesity. About 90 percent of all diabetics are Type II and weight loss and diet changes usually resolve the problem without the use of medi-cation. Black cumin can assist in this process.

The case of a fifty-eight-year-old woman who suffered from Type II diabetes, the so-called old age sugar, is typical. She had high blood-pressure and was overweight. In the case of adult onset diabe-tes, weight loss alone often alleviates the problem. Only in the rare cases is medication necessary to supplement insulin levels. Her doctor started by establishing a strict diet for her, and advised her to lose twenty pounds. At first the pounds disappeared as planned. Then, however, she reached a point at which the weight loss stopped. While her blood-sugar level had fallen, it did not seem possible to normalize it without the use of medication.

As she began to despair, the woman read in the paper about the effectiveness of black cumin oil therapy. She bought black cumin oil in capsules and started the basic treatment with the recommended dose of two capsules three times a day. In addition, she took a tablespoon of a special recipe of black cumin powder, elecampane (Inula helenium), *wild marjoram* (Origanum vulgare), *and finely ground crabapple peels before each meal.*

After three weeks her blood-sugar level had been reduced significantly, and her weight loss picked up again. The black cumin oil also had a positive influence on the metabolism and digestion of the patient. After another three weeks, her blood-sugar level was almost back to normal.

What You Can Do for Diabetes

Most Type II diabetics can normalize their elevated blood-sugar values by losing weight. Furthermore, a balanced diet that is low in carbohydrates is recommended. According to the latest scientific reports, foods with sugar are no longer prohibited but an excessively sugary diet should be avoided. And the annoying counting of calories and bread units seems to be outmoded as well.

Because diabetes can also be caused by food allergies, a healthy immune system is very important for all those with sugar problems. New research results from U.S. scientists suggest that in these cases black cumin oil can lower blood-sugar levels by strengthening the immune system.

Application for Diabetes

In the case of *diabetes mellitus* the basic treatment, which consists of 2 capsules or 25 drops of black cumin oil 3 times a day, is recommended. This treatment should be used for at least 4 weeks and can be continued indefinitely.

Caution: Diabetes is a serious illness, and although black cumin can help to resolve the
condition without synthetic drugs, you should
not self-treat. During black cumin therapy it is
essential to remain under the care of a doctor
so that blood-sugar levels can be monitored.
With some patients, these levels fall so dramatically that they can end up being too low.

SPECIAL RECIPE FOR DIABETES

1 cup (227 g) black cumin seeds
1 cup (227 g) elecampane (*Inula helenium*)
1 cup (227 g) wild marjoram (*Origanum vulgare*)
1 cup (227 g) crabapple peels

Grind and combine all the herbs and place them in a
bowl. Chop the crabapple peels, spread them on a cookie
sheet, cover with cheesecloth, and let them dry for a day.
Then grind them up finely as well and mix with the other
ingredients. Store the powder in a dark glass container in
a cool and dry place.

Take 1 tablespoon (15 g) of this mixture about 15
minutes before each meal. Continue this treatment for 4
weeks and then slowly reduce the dosage as the blood-
sugar level stabilizes.

EARACHES

Earache (*otitis media*) results from inflammation or infection of
the middle ear and is often preceded by an upper respiratory
infection, such as a cold or the flu. Respiratory allergies can

also promote ear infections by causing prolonged nasal congestion. Children suffer from ear infections especially frequently since the canal from the throat to the middle ear is shorter and wider in children than it is in adults. Harmful pathogens thus have an easier time getting to these sensitive areas of the ear.

Healing Ear Canal Infections

Because black cumin fights infections, it is well suited for the treatment of ear infections. Apply a few drops of pure black cumin oil into the ear canal with an eye dropper and massage a bit of oil behind the ear. Strengthen your immune system by eating foods high in vitamin C to cure every cold completely, before the infection is transferred to the ear. Quit or at least cut down on smoking.

EAR SALVE

2 tablespoons (30 ml) black cumin oil
2 tablespoons (30 g) finely ground black cumin seeds

Carefully heat the black cumin oil in a pan over the stove. Mix the ground black cumin seeds with the oil. Allow the mixture to cool.

Apply the salve 3 times a day to the outside ear canal. This recipe also helps for sinusitis and colds.

EYE STRAIN

Working for long periods of time on the computer, reading in low light, or driving on long trips strains the eye muscles, causing redness, burning, and tearing or, alternately, dryness.

In addition, unknown or uncorrected eye problems can precipitate eye strain. Chronic dryness of the eyes or retina or eyelid infections is a disorder that may be caused by pathogens, allergic reactions, or environmental toxins, so if the condition persists, be sure to consult your health care practitioner.

In addition to using black cumin compresses to relieve the symptoms of eye strain, take practical measures to reduce its occurrence. If you spend a lot of time working in front of a computer screen, position the screen so that natural light as well as artificial light come from the left (this applies to right-handed people; the inverse applies to left-handed people). Take frequent breaks throughout the day to close your eyes and rest them for a few moments, and every half hour focus on a distant point for a minute or two. And decrease your television consumption!

The antihistaminic qualities of black cumin oil can alleviate the soreness and pain caused by eye strain. Apply black cumin oil to your temples before going to bed or try a black cumin compress.

BLACK CUMIN EYE COMPRESS

1 tablespoon (15 g) black cumin seeds, roughly crushed
1 cup (240 ml) water
2 cotton washcloths

Boil the crushed black cumin seeds briefly in water, and then let them sit for 10 minutes. Soak the washcloths in the solution and then wring one out. Lie down and place the moist cloth on your closed eyes for about 10 minutes. When one cloth becomes cool, replace it in the pan and use the other one. Repeat for 30 minutes or until you feel relief.

FLATULENCE

The most common causes for flatulence are an unhealthy diet, lack of exercise, stress, and depression. When meals are not properly digested, gases accumulate in the intestines and cause discomfort. Flatulence is often a sign of intolerance of a certain food or of a damaged intestinal flora. Sometimes the intestines are unable to digest food completely due to illnesses (infection of the stomach's mucous membrane, infection of the pancreas, or irritation of the intestines) or disruptions such as diarrhea.

Recipe for Digestion Problems

The regulation of digestion is one of the most popular applications for black cumin in the Orient. In cases of chronic flatulence, eat 1 tablespoon of finely ground black cumin seeds each morning and then drink 1 glass of hot water sweetened with molasses or honey. In addition, take 2 black cumin capsules or 25 drops of black cumin oil 3 times a day.

BLACK CUMIN JUICE FOR FLATULENCE

16 ounces (480 ml) apple cider vinegar
1 cup (227 g) finely ground black cumin seeds
8 ounces (240 ml) black cumin oil

Heat the apple cider vinegar to about 130°F (50°C) and mix in the ground black cumin seeds. Add the liquid black cumin oil and let the liquid cool.

Take 1 tablespoon (15 ml), preferably at room temperature, 3 times a day before meals.

T. W., forty-eight, often experienced severe gas pains after eating. Doctors were not able to identify a cause. T. W. took synthetic anti-flatulence medications but they were not effective.

He began taking two capsules of black cumin oil three times a day. In addition, he took black cumin juice for flatulence before meals. After a week, gas pains were significantly better, and after three weeks they were entirely gone.

FUNGAL INFECTIONS

The spread of fungal infections is alarming: they have increased by 30 percent over the past ten years. The modern diet and lifestyle have weakened the immune system to the point that once harmless fungi are now growing out of control. *Candida albicans*, a yeast fungus that normally lives in the digestive tract and in the vagina without causing problems, is a good example. Widespread antibiotic use accompanied by sugar-rich diets and birth control pills have allowed yeast to proliferate, and yeast overgrowth is now recognized as causing chronic candidiasis.

Candidiasis is characterized by fatigue, allergies and chemical sensitivities, immune dysfunction, depression, and digestive problems. Women are affected much more often than men. Antibiotic use is the number one risk factor, and stress, environmental toxins, and a weakened immune system increase the chances of being afflicted.

A Strong Immune System

Black cumin oil contains substances that strengthen the immune system and discourage the growth of fungi. The ingestion of 2 capsules or 25 drops of black cumin oil 3 times a day prevents the *Candida* fungi from spreading and weakens it so that it can be kept in check by the intestinal bacteria. A successful treatment combines an antifungal diet without simple sugars (meaning no white sugar, no refined pasta, no fresh fruits).

BLACK CUMIN TO PREVENT YEAST OVERGROWTH

16 ounces (480 ml) apple cider vinegar
1 cup (227 g) finely ground black cumin seeds
8 ounces (240 ml) black cumin oil

Bring the apple cider vinegar to a boil, and then add the black cumin powder. Let the mixture boil for 5 more minutes while stirring constantly. Mix in the black cumin oil and continue to stir. Remove from heat when it has the consistency of syrup. Store in a dark glass container in a cool place.

Take 1 tablespoon (15 ml) 3 times a day before meals.

GALLBLADDER PROBLEMS

The gallbladder is a small, pear-shaped sac near the liver that stores bile, a yellow or greenish fluid secreted by the liver to assist the body's processing of fats. Bile has a number of components, including bile salts, bilirubin, cholesterol, phospholipids, fatty acids, and other substances. A diet low in fiber and high in animal protein, among other things, can lead to the formation of gallstones by encouraging bile to become supersaturated with cholesterol. Recent studies indicate that food allergies may be at the core of some gallbladder distress. If the gallstones become large enough, they can restrict the flow of bile and cause pain and inflammation. Women are four times more likely to have gallstones than men. Other risk factors include obesity and middle age.

Regulating the Gall Flow Naturally

Black cumin encourages the gallbladder to flush out toxic deposits and to maintain proper bile flow. Take 1 or 2 capsules or 25 drops black cumin oil 3 times a day. Avoid fat-rich foods and animal protein; a vegetarian diet seems to protect against gallstone formation. Use marjoram frequently in cooking. Reduce consumption of alcohol and caffeine, since these burden the liver and affect the bile flow.

BLACK CUMIN FOR THE GALLBLADDER

$^1/_2$ teaspoon ($2^1/_2$ g) wild marjoram (*Origanum vulgare*)
8 ounces (240 ml) honey
1 tablespoon black cumin seeds

Chop the marjoram and mix it with the honey. Grind up the black cumin seeds and combine with the marjoram and honey to make a paste.

For chronic gallbladder problems, take 1 tablespoon (15 g) 2 times a day.

GUM INFECTIONS

Infected gums are red and painfully swollen and bleed under even slight pressure. The main cause is a buildup of layers of bacteria on the teeth and tartar. If the infection becomes constant, the gums recede. Bacteria then invade and attack the jaw until it can no longer hold the teeth.

Soothing Infectious Processes

Because of its antibacterial qualities, black cumin fights gum infections and strengthens the tissue. In addition to the treatment described below, gargling with black cumin oil has also proven successful. Swish 1 teaspoon of black cumin oil through the teeth for about 15 minutes so that it coats the gums and the mouth's mucous membranes. Spit out the oil afterward (do not swallow).

ANTI-INFECTION POWDER

1 tablespoon (15 g) black cumin seeds
1 tablespoon (15 g) anise
1 tablespoon (15 g) cloves

Grind together the black cumin, anise, and cloves, thoroughly mixing all ingredients.

Take 1 teaspoon (5 g) of this powder 3 times a day after brushing your teeth. Using your tongue, press the powder against your gums for a few seconds and then swallow. This application is also helpful for toothaches caused by infected wisdom teeth or cavities.

HEADACHES

Headaches can be caused by a wide variety of factors, and most do not signal a serious disease. The most common type of headache is the so-called tension headache. This type of headache usually consists of a steady, dull pain that spreads from the back of the head or the forehead to the entire head. Tension headaches are often described as feeling like one's head is being gripped in a vise, and generally occur in response to poor posture and excessive stress. Migraines are characterized by throbbing, pounding, sharp pain. Often the pain occurs on one side only and is accompanied by such symptoms as vomiting and hypersensitivity to light and noise. Migraines can be caused by changes in the weather, hormones, or stress.

Headaches themselves are not an illness, but rather the symptom of various illnesses. There is a difference between independent headaches (such as the tension headache) and those that are caused by illnesses such as infections or disruptions in the metabolism. Headaches can have many causes, and it is important to find the specific cause in each case before deciding on the proper treatment.

Getting Rid of Persistent Headaches

Black cumin is especially helpful for headaches caused by hormones. The recommended dosage is 2 capsules or 20–25 drops of black cumin oil 3 times a day. Before starting this treatment, however, you should consult your doctor, especially if headaches are accompanied by vision problems, dizziness, and partial paralysis of limbs, or if they start after physical exertion or occur for the first time past the age of forty.

RECIPE FOR HEADACHES

1 cup (227 g) black cumin seeds
1 cup (227 g) anise
1 cup (227 g) cloves

Grind all the herbs together until they form a fine powder. Place the powder in a dark glass container and store in a cool, dry place.

Take 1 teaspoon (5 g) 2 times a day, before breakfast and lunch. Chew the powder thoroughly and swallow it. Do not wash it down with water. Allow it to be absorbed by the mouth's mucous membrane.

HEMORRHOIDS

Chronic constipation, severe physical exertion, lack of exercise, and a predominantly sedentary lifestyle favor the onset of hemorrhoids. These knotty veins cause itching and burning sensations in the anus. In the later stages, there can be cramps and stinging pain as well as bleeding during bowel movements. Black cumin regulates the digestion and also has antihistaminic effects, which alleviate these symptoms noticeably. For the treatment of hemorrhoids prepare a cream using the ash of burned black cumin seeds.

Pay attention to diet and increase consumption of high-fiber foods. If you are not used to eating high-fiber foods, build up slowly to avoid aggravating the problem. Drink 2 quarts of water a day to keep the digestive system working smoothly and avoid strongly spiced dishes as well as alcohol. Exercise regularly and wear only cotton underwear.

BLACK CUMIN HEMORRHOID CREAM

2 tablespoons (30 g) black cumin seeds
1 tablespoon (15 ml) black cumin oil

Roast the black cumin seeds in an iron pan on the stove until they are burned. Let the seeds cool, and then grind them into a powder. Add the black cumin oil to make a spreadable cream.

Carefully clean the anus 2 times a day and after every bowel movement. Pat dry and gently apply the cream.

If the hemorrhoids do not respond to this treatment within 4 weeks, consult your health care practitioner. Severe cases require medical treatment.

H. W., a forty-three-year-old male, had suffered from hemorrhoids since childhood. He occasionally experienced bright red rectal bleeding and often used over-the-counter cortisone creams to treat the itching. The hemorrhoids were aggravated by his obesity, constipation, and sedentary lifestyle. He had already had one hemorrhoid surgically cauterized and was searching for a way to resolve the problem without further operations.

H. W. began taking two teaspoons (ten grams) of black cumin oil before each meal. Improvement was apparent after only a few weeks, and after three years of black cumin therapy the patient is no longer bothered by hemorrhoids.

HIGH BLOOD PRESSURE

The medical term for high blood pressure is *hypertension*. The normal blood pressure for an adult is 120 (systolic)/80 (diastolic). Doctors consider blood pressure to be mildly elevated when it measures at more than 140–160/95–104 for an extended period of time. High blood pressure causes no pain but in the long run weakens the blood vessels because of constant strain. This paves the way for serious illnesses such as heart attacks, heart disease, or strokes.

In many cases, high blood pressure can be prevented or reversed by changing one's diet and lifestyle. The drugs most often prescribed for the condition often have bothersome side effects, and new research shows that they do not reduce the incidence of heart attack or heart disease. While anyone currently taking high blood pressure medication should not discontinue it without consulting his or her physician, chances are good that the condition can be resolved without synthetic drugs.

Some lifestyle issues related to high blood pressure include coffee consumption, alcohol intake, lack of aerobic exercise, smoking, and stress. Dietary risk factors include being overweight, having a low-fiber, high-sodium, high-fat diet; and being deficient in vitamin C, calcium, magnesium, and potassium. Current studies point to a number of foods that may help lower blood pressure: celery, garlic, onions, cold-water fish, beans and grains, and green leafy vegetables. A holistic program that combines a heart-healthy diet, relaxation and stress-reducing techniques, and aerobic exercise three times per week can have an extremely positive effect on blood pressure.

Black Cumin for Healthier Veins

Studies indicate that black cumin can contribute to blood vessel health as well when incorporated into a general program of diet and lifestyle changes. Add 5 drops of black cumin oil to a warm drink 4 or 5 times a day and drink it slowly. Black cumin syrup (see page 39) may also be effective in lowering blood pressure.

IMPOTENCE

For many men, a bout with impotence—or erectile dysfunction as it is often called—shakes the foundation of their self-esteem and identity. They may avoid bringing the problem to the attention of their local doctor because the issue is too sensitive or embarrassing to discuss. Some men even hide the problem from their own partner, feigning fatigue or working late to avoid going to bed at the same time. However, things are changing. Recent media attention to the topic of erectile dysfunction is beginning to change the stigma of the condition, and more men are realizing that seeking help can be the first step toward resolving the issue.

When doctors today speak of erectile dysfunction they emphasize that the problem stems from inadequate blood flow, not a lack of "potency." The influx of blood to the penis during the phase of sexual excitement is not sufficient to cause or maintain an erection. If an erection does occur, usually it either is not strong enough or does not last long enough to permit intercourse. Doctors used to assume that the vast majority of erectile problems had a psychological basis. According to today's knowledge, however, a number of physical factors can cause short-term impotence, including:

- Smoking
- Disruptions in the hormonal system
- Disruptions of the metabolism
- Lack of exercise
- Obesity
- Rheumatic illnesses
- High blood pressure
- Environmental toxins
- Alcohol or drugs
- Stress

Black Cumin to Enhance Potency

Because black cumin can help to resolve some of the underlying causes of erectile dysfunction, it is a powerful ally in restoring sexual performance. Its healing properties, when combined with changes in diet and lifestyle, can renew virility without drugs. Black cumin increases overall well-being while enhancing the production of body fluids and male hormones and rejuvenating blood circulation.

The recommended dosage is 2 capsules or 25 drops of black cumin oil 3 times a day. Eastern medicine also recommends the following recipe to amplify these good effects.

BLACK CUMIN FOR POTENCY

1 cup (227 g) black cumin seeds
1 cup (227 g) elecampane (*Inula helenium*)
1 tablespoon (15 g) wild marjoram (*Origanum vulgare*)
2 tablespoons (30 g) fenugreek

Finely grind all ingredients, put them in a bowl, and mix thoroughly.

Mix 1 tablespoon (15 g) of this mixture with honey each morning and take about 15 minutes before breakfast. Do not swallow immediately but let it melt slowly in the mouth. The treatment takes 6 weeks. After ingestion, drink 1 glass of whole milk mixed with malt in a 1:1 ratio. Eat a lot of fresh fruit. And exercise in the mornings!

INSECT BITES

Mosquito bites are generally harmless since the redness and swelling fade quickly if you do not scratch them. The stings from bees and wasps are worse; they lead to noticeable swelling and tenderness.

You can protect yourself against insects effectively by burning black cumin seeds. If an open fire is not available, a pan heated on a stove until the seeds are roasted will have the same effect. It is especially effective to burn the black cumin together with incense in an incense burner. This not only smells pleasant, but also keeps insects away—and allows you to enjoy the summer evening in peace.

BLACK CUMIN INSECT REPELLANT

1 tablespoon (15 g) black cumin seeds
1 tablespoon (15 g) powdered incense

Spread the black cumin evenly on the bottom of a cast-iron pan. Sprinkle the incense on top. Let both roast slowly either over an open fire (barbecue pit), or on the stove set at the lowest heat.

Stay within the range of the aromatic mixture.

For stings on the throat or in the event of allergic reaction (shortness of breath, dizziness, severe swelling), go to the nearest emergency room immediately. Doctors will administer an injection of epinephrine to prevent allergic (anaphylactic) shock.

INSOMNIA

Insomnia affects up to 30 percent of the population in any given year. Insomnia is characterized by difficulty in falling asleep or in remaining asleep. About half of all problems with insomnia stem from psychological factors such as depression or anxiety. Other causes include stress, certain medications, lack of exercise, and high caffeine intake. The first step in resolving insomnia is to pinpoint the cause or causes and then address each issue individually.

To support better sleeping patterns, try to set aside time 3 days a week for 20 minutes of aerobic exercise. Eliminate or at least cut down on your daily caffeine consumption. It is also helpful to plan a relaxing evening ritual: make a list of what you need to take care of the following day so your mind will be clear and ready for sleep and take a warm bath or shower or listen to soft music for 30 minutes before bedtime. A dark, quiet, and well-ventilated room as well as a sufficiently large bed with a good, firm mattress set the right conditions for a good night's sleep. Do not take naps during the daytime.

In the East, black cumin has long been used to promote a deep, restful sleep and a calm mind. The best way to reap black cumin's benefits is to prepare a strong decoction: boil a few tablespoons of black cumin seeds in 2 cups of water for 30 to 45 minutes. Strain and drink. Drinking nerve tea during the day instead of coffee or black tea can help too.

NERVE TEA

1 cup (227 g) black cumin seeds
1 quart (1 l) water

Crush the black cumin seeds and place in a prewarmed teapot. Boil the water and pour over the seeds. Let the tea steep, covered, for 10 minutes, and then strain it. Keep the tea warm during the day in a thermos.

Drink the tea throughout the day, beginning with 1 cup in the morning before breakfast. Take the last cup 1 or 2 hours before going to bed.

INTESTINAL AILMENTS

Heartburn, feeling overly full, vomiting, diarrhea, and constipation are usually the result of a bad diet, harmful fungi in the intestines, or severe psychological strain. They can also be symptoms of a more serious condition.

The active ingredients contained in black cumin balance the intestinal tract thus resolve intestinal discomfort. Take 1 capsule or 20–25 drops of black cumin oil 3 times a day. If problems recur frequently, continue the treatment with black cumin for up to 3 weeks.

Eastern medicine recommends the ingestion of lukewarm black cumin milk for acute intestinal ailments. The milk also has a soothing effect on the damaged mucous membrane of the stomach.

BLACK CUMIN MILK

8 ounces (240 ml) milk
2 tablespoons (30 g) black cumin oil
1 tablespoon (15 ml) honey

Slowly heat the milk over medium heat. Remove from the stove and add the black cumin oil. Stir in the honey, combining all ingredients thoroughly.

Take 1 tablespoon (15 ml) 3 times a day before meals.

B. M., forty-two, experienced abdominal cramps that were not related to meals. The family physician was unable to find any logical causes. She began taking two capsules of black cumin oil three times a day, and after only two weeks the cramps subsided. She continues to take black cumin oil daily and remains pain free.

JOINT PAINS

Joint pains are caused either by a worn-down joint or by infection of a joint. In infectious joint rheumatism, autoimmune processes play a large role. For unknown reasons, the immune system not only reacts to foreign substances in the joint, but attacks the body's own substances as well. Typical symptoms are stiffness in the morning and prolonged swelling of the joints, pain or pressure during movement, as well as rheumatic knots.

Preventing Infections of the Joints

An autoimmune reaction can be regulated by taking 1 or 2 capsules or 20–25 drops of black cumin oil 3 times a day. Apply black cumin joint cream as needed for relief. Ailments that are caused by a worn-down joint (due either to illness or old age) cannot be cured with the application of black cumin but can at least be alleviated.

Strengthening Connective Tissue

To tighten and rejuvenate the connecting tissue you should take 2 capsules or 25 drops black cumin oil 3 times a day. In addition, take a multivitamin and 1 gram vitamin C. Black cumin oil and apple cider vinegar mixtures have proven successful for rejuvenating weak connective tissue as well.

BLACK CUMIN JOINT CREAM

2 tablespoons (30 ml) black cumin oil
2 tablespoons (30 g) freshly ground black cumin seeds

Place the black cumin oil in a small pot and warm it over low heat. Add the black cumin powder to make a spreadable cream. Allow the mixture to cool, and store it in a dark glass container in a cool, dry place.

Apply the cream to the affected joints 2 times a day. For joint infections, the cream should be as cool as possible. For joint inflammation, the cream should be warmed up before being applied.

KIDNEY STONES

Kidney stones are usually caused by an unbalanced diet that contains too much fat and protein and not enough fiber. Stress, lack of exercise, and a hereditary predisposition also are factors. The substances contained in the urine are not excreted sufficiently and deposits begin to build up. Kidney stones can cause painful cramping that extends around the bladder area and the back. Common symptoms once the stone becomes dislodged include vomiting, distension of the abdomen, chills, and fever.

Quick Help for Acute Pains

Black cumin soothes the pain caused by kidney stones, relaxing the cramping and preventing infection. For mild cramping,

1 tablespoon of black cumin seeds taken before breakfast provides relief.

Black cumin syrup is another effective remedy (see page 39). Take 1 tablespoon (15 ml) before breakfast for 20 days.

Kidney poultices have also proven successful: heat 2 tablespoons olive oil, mix in 2 tablespoons finely ground black cumin, and let sit for 15 minutes. Then apply the mixture to a cotton cloth and place the cloth on the kidney area. To keep the warmth in, wrap the area with plastic wrap and cover with a large towel or old blanket. Leave the poultice on until it cools. Repeat as necessary.

PREMENSTRUAL SYNDROME

Premenstrual syndrome (PMS) is characterized by uncomfortable symptoms that begin a week or two before menstruation and recur from cycle to cycle. Symptoms often include headache, low energy, tension, depression, irritability, breast tenderness, water retention, backache, and abdominal cramps. Studies have established that the physical causes of PMS that stem from multiple factors, including hormone imbalance, stress, depression, and nutritional deficiencies.

Black cumin has been used as a traditional remedy for menstrual complaints for hundreds of years, and now scientists are beginning to understand the mechanism of this useful herb. When used in concert with a healthy, low-fat diet and regular exercise, black cumin can assist in normalizing the absorption of essential fatty acids, which is disturbed in women who suffer from PMS. By regulating the metabolism, black cumin can help prevent PMS.

Drink 1 cup of black cumin tea (see page 36) 2 times a day

beginning on day 14 of your cycle and continuing through menstruation. To relieve cramping, try massaging warm black cumin skin oil into the abdomen (see page 71). Drinking 2 cups of black cumin tea a day for up to 6 months can also prevent some of the uncomfortable symptoms of menopause.

For Women Taking Birth Control Pills

The synthetic hormones in the birth control pill change the environment of a woman's genital tract, and women who take the Pill may be more susceptible to vaginitis. Women can combat this by taking 2 capsules or 25 drops of black cumin oil 3 times a day to keep their immune systems strong. Taking a multivitamin is also a good idea. Pill use increases the body's need for vitamins C, B_2 (riboflavin), B_{12}, B_6 (pyridoxine), and folic acid.

SKIN AILMENTS

Black cumin oil can be applied externally to treat a number of skin conditions, including infections, eczema, bruises and sprains, skin parasites, skin fungi, neurodematitis, and psoriasis. Because black cumin oil soothes itching and prevents infection, it is the perfect way to treat these disorders without resorting to synthetic drugs.

For the treatment of these ailments, liquid black cumin oil is applied to the affected area either straight or mixed with other healing substances. One easy recipe that soothes itching and speeds healing combines black cumin with apple cider vinegar.

SOOTHING BLACK CUMIN SKIN CREAM

2 cups (480 ml) apple cider vinegar
1 cup (227 g) finely ground black cumin seeds
1 cup (227 g) cornstarch

Heat the apple cider vinegar and add the ground black cumin seeds. Bring to a boil and then add the cornstarch. Blend thoroughly and remove from heat. Let the cream cool. Store in a dark glass container in a cool, dry place.

Apply the cream 2 times a day to the affected area. The cream is most effective if it is applied before going to bed. The cream is especially effective on external fungal infections.

Eczema

Eczema is a common skin disorder characterized by an itchy rash that may also be patchy, dry, thick, and bumpy. Scratching the affected area spreads the bacteria on the skin and can lead to serious infections. Eczema occurs most often in people with allergies and usually runs in the family. There are several types of eczema, including atopic (allergic) eczema, neurodermatitis (discussed below), and contact dermatitis.

Dietary changes can have a positive effect on the incidence and severity of outbreaks for those suffering from atopic eczema. The most common food culprits are milk, eggs, peanuts, fish, soy, wheat, and citrus. Contact dermatitis can be eliminated by avoiding contact with the substance causing the reaction.

Treating eczema with black cumin oil often leads to surprisingly quick results. Treatment combines internal application (2 capsules or 25 drops of black cumin oil 3 times a day) with external application. For local treatment, applying ozonized black cumin oil directly to the rash is most successful. (Ozonized black cumin oil is bubbled through a chemically altered form of oxygen for an extended period of time.)

Black cumin cream (see page 70) offers relief if applied to the affected skin area several times a day.

Neurodermatitis

Neurodermatitis is a severe, chronic form of eczema. The main symptom is an itchy crust that forms on the body, especially the neck, wrists, elbows, and the backs of the knees. Children affected by neurodermatitis often have crusts that appear on the scalp.

Its beginnings are favored by an allergic predisposition, although psychological factors are believed to play a role in its outbreak as well. Almost 20 percent of patients also suffer from asthma, and more than 10 percent suffer from hay fever. Neurodermatitis is not contagious.

Black cumin is an effective treatment for neurodermatitis. It soothes the itch, stabilizes the immune system, and supports the healing of the infected skin areas. Take 2 capsules or 25 drops of black cumin oil 3 times a day.

Applying black cumin skin oil (see below) externally can relieve itching and irritation.

BLACK CUMIN SKIN OIL

3 tablespoons (45 ml) black cumin oil
3 tablespoons (45 g) finely ground black cumin seeds

Carefully heat the black cumin oil in a pan over medium heat. Add the ground black cumin seeds to the oil and blend thoroughly. Filter the mixture and allow it to cool. Store in a dark glass container in a cool, dry place.

Apply the oil to the affected skin areas 3 times a day. The cooler the oil is when you apply it, the more soothing it will be.

Fungal Infections

If you discover red lesions on your skin with itchy, flaky pimples, you may be dealing with a fungal infection. You should consult your doctor for a diagnosis because proper treatment depends in part on the type of fungus causing the infection. Fungal infections are very contagious, and warm, wet places such as public baths or locker rooms, saunas, and hot tubs offer ideal growing conditions.

Doctors often prescribe cortisone for this condition, which is effective but has a number of side effects. Black cumin cream (see page 70) provides a healthy, effective alternative. To support the external application, you should also ingest 2 capsules or 25 drops black cumin oil 3 times a day. You can expect the rash and itchiness to disappear within 1 week.

W. U., a six-year-old male, had recurrent fungal infections on the torso and legs that did not respond to antimycotic medications. He often took antibiotics for other infections, which may have made him more susceptible to fungal infections.

He took one capsule of black cumin oil three times a day for six months. After four weeks, the infected areas had cleared up completely. He has not had any recurrences. In addition, he has not needed antibiotics for any other infections.

Parasites

In spite of careful hygiene, many people today occasionally get skin parasites. Often people bring them home from vacations, and children contract lice and scabies at school or in daycare centers. For centuries in the East, black cumin has been applied externally to kill parasites safely.

Lice

Human lice (*Pediculidae*) are wingless, light gray insects one to three millimeters in length. They stick to the hair, feed on human blood, and carry diseases. One head-louse can lay up to 100 eggs. Their development takes about three to four weeks. Head-lice are passed on through physical contact and cause severe itching. The slightly larger clothes-louse is more dangerous since it can pass on borrelia, bacterial pathogens.

When you have lice, only careful hygiene will help: wash your entire body thoroughly and disinfect the affected skin areas. In addition, wash all clothes and bedding and vacuum the mattress and other soft furnishings. Massage the basic recipe (see next page) thoroughly into the hair and let it dry for at least 15 minutes in the sun or under a hair dryer. Allow it to stay in the hair for at least 4 hours and then wash it out using a mild shampoo. Repeat daily. In most cases this treatment is effective within 1 week.

Scabies

Scabies is a contagious skin disease caused by the tiny, spiderlike itch mite (*Sarcoptes scabiei*). The female digs a burrow under the skin to lay eggs, which hatch three to five days later. The young mites emerge to mate on the skin's surface, and then the life cycle continues. The main symptom of scabies is intense itching, most often occurring in skin folds between the fingers, under the arms, and on the wrists, elbows, breasts, penis, and lower back.

To treat scabies with black cumin massage the basic recipe on the affected skin areas and leave it on for about 4 hours. Then wash the treatment off with a mild, unscented natural soap. Rub pure black cumin oil on afterward. Continue the treatment for at least 1 week.

BASIC RECIPE FOR SKIN PARASITES

1 cup (227 g) finely ground black cumin seeds
8 ounces (240 ml) apple cider vinegar

In a bowl, blend the ground black cumin seeds with the apple cider vinegar and let the mixture sit for about 10 minutes. Then filter the mixture through a cloth, squeezing out as much moisture as possible. Place the black cumin sediment remaining in the cloth in the sun to allow as much fluid as possible to evaporate. The resulting mass should be thick and almost dry.

Apply the paste to the affected skin areas or the hair and allow it to dry for at least 15 minutes. Allow it to be absorbed for 4 hours, and then rinse off with warm water.

Psoriasis

Psoriasis is a skin disease characterized by thick, raised, red patches covered with silvery white scales. The patches result when the outer layers of skin divide much more rapidly than normal, although the causes are unknown. The patches may burn, crack, and bleed, and there is no permanent cure for the condition. The areas most affected are the knees and elbows but the patches may affect any area of the body. The predisposition to psoriasis is hereditary and is amplified by psychological strain.

Conventional treatment of psoriasis consists of cortisone therapy or the application of coal tars. Fortunately, black cumin oil offers an effective natural alternative. To stimulate healing from the inside, take 2 capsules or 25 drops of black cumin oil 3 times a day.

In addition, keep the infected skin covered with a layer of black cumin skin oil at all times (see page 71).

A vacation at the ocean or near the Dead Sea can have marvelous healing effects. If world travel is not an option, you can also purchase Dead Sea salts for the bath in a pharmacy or health food store.

S. S., fifty-six, had been troubled since childhood by a severe case of psoriasis. Her back, forearms, calves, and scalp were especially afflicted. She had tried steroid therapy as well as a vacation to the Dead Sea, but the problem remained the same.

She began treating the scaly patches topically with black cumin oil before a session of light therapy and after a bath. She also took two capsules of black cumin three times a day. This treatment significantly reduced the scaliness of the affected areas.

TUMORS

A tumor may be harmless or malignant. A harmless growth is an isolated growth of new tissue. While it can press on nerves and neighboring organs, it will not extend into any other organs. In contrast, a malignant growth (cancer) spreads into neighboring tissues or organs and forms new growths (metastases). Tumor cells look for a weak spot in the organism and attempt to spread out from there. They are successful only if the immune system has been compromised.

Cancer Prevention with Black Cumin

Black cumin oil plays an important role in tumor treatment. It stimulates the production of bone marrow and immune cells and increases the production of interferon, a protein that fights the growth of harmful microorganisms. For the prevention of tumors, take 2 capsules or 25 drops of black cumin oil 3 times a day for 6 months.

The following recipe for tumor prevention may also help the body fight off unhealthy cellular changes.

BLACK CUMIN FOR TUMOR PREVENTION

2 tablespoons (30 ml) black cumin oil
2 tablespoons (30 g) finely ground black cumin seeds
1 tablespoon (15 g) royal jelly

Slightly heat the black cumin oil in a pan, and mix it with the ground black cumin seeds. Mix in the royal jelly and remove from heat. Let the syrup cool and store in a dark glass container in a cool, dry place.

Take 1 teaspoon (5 g) 3 times a day before meals. Continue the application for 6 weeks, and then reduce the dosage to 1 teaspoon (5 g) 2 times a day.

WOUNDS

Wounds or tissue injuries are usually the result of leisure activities, especially athletic ones. Wounds heal in several phases. First, a crust forms to close off the wound. A little later the so-called granulation tissue forms under this crust; this new tissue is lined with blood vessels. Finally, a scar forms. Wounds heal more quickly if the tissue has a good blood circulation. That is why disruptions in metabolism often retard the healing of wounds.

Caring for Open Wounds

Because of its antibacterial qualities, black cumin was used in ancient Egypt for the treatment of open wounds. Black cumin discourages infections and accelerates the healing process.

Clean the wound under running water. Apply black cumin salve to a clean linen cloth and tie gently to the injured area. Change the bandage daily. Seek medical attention if redness or swelling persists because the wound may be infected.

WOUND SALVE

3 tablespoons (45 g) finely ground black cumin seeds
2 tablespoons (30 ml) black cumin oil
1 tablespoon (15 ml) apple cider vinegar

Roast the ground black cumin seeds in a cast-iron pan until the powder is blackened. Combine with the black cumin oil and apple cider vinegar. The resulting mixture should have the consistency of a salve.

After washing the wound with soap and water, dab the area with a bit of apple cider vinegar on a cotton ball. Allow the area to dry completely and apply the salve.

> **Caution: Deep or puncture wounds require immediate medical attention.**

FOUR

Black Cumin for Healthy Skin, Hair, and Nails

BLACK CUMIN'S REPUTATION as a healing plant extends to its usefulness in a variety of beauty preparations. Black cumin provides the body with important polyunsaturated fatty acids. Because of its ideal combination of active ingredients, black cumin's positive effects on the skin, hair, and nails reach deep beneath the surface, healing and preventing the damaging effects of our stressful modern lifestyles.

While one can find a large selection of beauty products that contain black cumin in Egypt, such products are hard to find in our stores. However, it is easy and economical to make your own oils, creams, scrubs, and masks at home. Making your own concoctions also allows you to avoid the synthetic chemicals and preservatives found in commercial products.

CARING FOR YOUR SKIN

The skin is the body's largest organ. It weighs between seven and ten pounds and would cover about twenty square feet if spread out flat. The epidermis, the skin's outer layer, constantly renews itself with cells growing from inner layers. The skin does indeed "breathe," allowing oxygen to enter the body and excreting toxins along with perspiration. The skin is heavily influenced by pollution, nutrition, and stress, so lifestyle plays a major role in whether you sport glowing and clear cheeks or a splotchy, tender face (see page 31 for acne remedies).

To nourish your skin effectively and naturally from the inside, place $1/2$ cup (114 g) of raisins in 8 ounces (240 ml) of black cumin oil and combine in a covered glass jar. Let the raisins steep in the oil for a few days. Take 1 tablespoon (15 ml) of the raisins together with the oil every day. You can also chew black cumin seeds together with raisins, or take black cumin capsules and eat a handful of raisins as a daily snack.

By the way, black cumin and raisins not only make your skin smooth and soft but also taste good and ensure fresh breath. You will no longer need to use mouthwash.

The following recipes will help your skin repair and renew itself.

Nourishing Facial Creams

Add a few drops of black cumin oil to your favorite facial cream, or make your own cream with the following recipe.

In a double boiler, gently heat $1^2/3$ cups (400 ml) black cumin oil with an equal amount of jojoba oil. Add $1/3$ ounce

(75 g) grated beeswax and slowly heat the mixture to 140°F (60°C), until the wax has melted. Thoroughly mix the ingredients and allow the mixture to cool. Store the cream in a glass jar and keep in a cool place.

Depending on personal preference and skin type, you can also add a few drops of essential oil to your cream. For sensitive skin, add sandalwood, rose, or camellia. For troubled skin, use a mixture of peppermint oil and arnica extract. Camphor, lavender, sage, and tea tree oils will balance oily skin. Good additions for dry skin are bergamot, grapefruit, and ylang ylang.

Cleansing Facial Scrub

Exfoliating once a week allows you to remove the buildup of dead skin and reveals the fresh new skin underneath. Crush 1 tablespoon (15 g) of black cumin seeds and mix a few drops of black cumin oil into the powder until it forms a paste. Apply to the face with circular motions and leave it on for about 10 minutes. Rinse your face with warm water. (If you have oily skin, wash your face with soap and water.)

You can also try using this cleansing scrub on your elbows, knees, and feet in the bath or shower to soften and condition the skin.

Soothing Facial Mask

Mix 1 egg yolk with 1 teaspoon (5 ml) each of black cumin oil and wheat germ oil. Add a splash of lemon juice and a little bit of honey. Mix all ingredients thoroughly. Apply to the face and leave on for 30 minutes. Wash off with warm water.

Restoring Firm, Elastic Skin

To restore a supple texture to damaged skin, take 2 capsules or 25 drops black cumin oil 3 times a day. In addition, to be sure you are getting the important nutrients that feed your skin, take a multivitamin with zinc. Adding 1 or 2 spoonfuls of black cumin oil to the bath 2 times a week will also revitalize tired skin.

Refreshing Body Oil

Black cumin nourishes the skin and stimulates blood circulation. It is thus an excellent basis for body oils.

To create your own body oil, mix an equal amount of black cumin oil with wheat germ oil; use modest amounts to prevent the oils from becoming rancid before you can use them. Add a few drops of an essential oil according to your skin type or fragrance preference. For oily skin, try juniper or rosemary. For dry skin use geranium, orange, or patchouli. For mature skin, add lavender or ylang ylang.

Smooth on a few drops of the body oil after bathing, while your skin is still damp.

HEALTHY HAIR AND NAILS

Like skin cells, hair and skin cells move upward as new ones form underneath. When the cells reach the surface, they are cut off from their supply of nourishment and form a hard protein called keratin. The hair and nails you actually see comprise layers of dead cells that must be treated gently to prevent breakage.

Many factors influence the growth and texture of hair and nails—age, diet, general health, and seasonal changes as well as pollution, overexposure to the sun or chlorinated water, smoking, and alcohol consumption. Personal habits or grooming practices also influence the condition of our hair and nails. It is difficult to maintain strong nails if you use chemical cleaning products every day without wearing gloves. Even brushing your hair with a synthetic hair brush can be damaging. Thus shiny hair and strong nails require a healthy lifestyle with minimal exposure to toxins—a good diet, exercise, and plenty of pure water. Fortunately, black cumin can help repair and prevent damage to both.

Full Bodied, Shiny Hair

Black cumin oil nourishes the scalp and the roots of the hair and makes hair noticeably stronger and softer. For healthy hair, or to revitalize dry or damaged hair, taking black cumin oil internally is very effective. The dose is 2 capsules or 25 drops of black cumin oil 3 times a day.

Diet can make a significant difference in the health of your hair. Zinc is an essential vitamin for the health of hair and skin. Foods rich in zinc include beans, beef, bran, cantaloupe, cheese, clams, crab, fish, liver, milk, nuts, pork, raw sprouts, whole grains, and yogurt. Taking a daily mutivitamin that includes zinc and selenium, another vitamin that contributes to the elasticity of tissue, will ensure that your body has the essential nutrients to keep your hair healthy.

Repairing and Strengthening Hair

If you have dry, lusterless hair, mix a few drops of black cumin oil in with your shampoo and apply the shampoo as usual.

For very dry or damaged hair, a more intensive treatment is more successful. Try this deep conditioning treatment first daily and later once a week, until the texture of the hair shows improvement. This may reduce flaking caused by a dry scalp.

Combine 2 tablespoons (30 g) finely ground black cumin seeds, 2 tablespoons (30 ml) garden rocket (*eruca vesicaria*) juice, 1 tablespoon (15 ml) apple cider vinegar, and 8 ounces (240 ml) of cold-pressed olive oil. Massaging this conditioning treatment into the scalp for at least 5 minutes. Pay special attention to the ends of the hair as well if the hair is damaged. Leave the mixture in the hair for 20 to 30 minutes.

It is especially nice to apply this conditioner during a bath; cover the hair with a plastic shower cap, wrap the head with a warm, moist towel, and relax while the oils soak into the hair shafts. Remove the conditioner by shampooing and rinsing the hair thoroughly.

Stronger Fingernails

Nails are a window to our internal health, indicating whether our diets and lifestyles need improvement and adjustment or whether we are on the right path. Black cumin oil can help nails become strong and smooth again. Take 2 capsules or 25 drops of black cumin oil 3 times a day.

You can also nourish nails by soaking your fingertips for 20 to 30 minutes in a small bowl of warm olive or wheat germ oil to which you've added 2 tablespoons (30 ml) of black cumin oil. A few drops of essential oil can be added for fragrance.

This treatment is especially effective if you massage the warm oils into the hands after soaking the nails for 30 minutes. Pull on a pair of clean cotton gloves and allow the oils to moisturize the hands and nails overnight. In the morning your hands will be soft and smooth.

Nails also require essential vitamins and minerals, so eating well and taking a multivitamin may yield results more quickly. If you have white spots on your nails, you may not be getting enough zinc (see page 82 for a list of foods rich in zinc).

FIVE

~~~

Black Cumin in the Kitchen

IT IS IMPOSSIBLE TO IMAGINE the cuisine of the Middle East without black cumin, and black cumin should be part of any healthy diet. Not only is it an incredible nutritional supplement, but the seeds are also a delicious spice. In this chapter you will find a wonderful range of recipes for introducing black cumin into your diet. But you don't need to use our recipes; simply follow the lead of Arab bakers and mix $1/_8$ pound (56 g) of black cumin seeds per pound (454 g) of flour into the dough of your favorite recipe, or apply a mixture of egg yolk and water to the top of the loaf and sprinkle with the seeds before baking.

SOUR RYE BREAD

$1/_2$ pound (227 g) wheat flour
1 pound (454 g) rye flour
1 teaspoon (5 g) salt

1 tablespoon (30 ml) black cumin oil

2 cups (480 ml) buttermilk

$^1/_2$ cup (114 g) butter

1 packet yeast

$^1/_2$ pound (227 g) natural sourdough starter

$^1/_4$ cup (60 ml) milk

3 tablespoons (45 g) black cumin seeds

Mix the ingredients into a dough that is not too sticky. Keep it in a warm place and let it rise to about twice its size. Add some flour, knead the dough again, and form it into a loaf. Cut slits in the surface, brush milk on top, and sprinkle with the black cumin seeds. Let the dough rise again. Then bake at 350°F (176°C) for 40 to 50 minutes.

BLACK CUMIN ROLLS

1 pound (454 g) wheat flour

1 pinch salt

$^1/_2$ cup (120 ml) milk

$^1/_4$ cup (60 ml) butter

1 packet yeast

1 teaspoon (5 g) sugar

2 tablespoons (30 g) black cumin seeds

Knead the ingredients into a dough. Keep dough in a warm place and let it rise to twice its size. Knead again, form into balls, and let them rise again on a buttered rack. Push a dent into each, brush with butter, and sprinkle with black cumin seeds. Bake the rolls at 350°F (176°C) for about 15 minutes.

CURLED ROLLS

1 pound (454 g) wheat flour

1 pinch salt

1$^1/_4$ cup (300 ml) milk

1 packet yeast

1 teaspoon (5 g) sugar

3 tablespoons (45 g) butter

1 egg yolk

2 tablespoons (30 g) black cumin seeds

Knead ingredients into soft dough, put it in a warm place, and let it rise. Knead again. Divide into 12 equal-sized pieces. Roll them out, then roll them up. Let them rise on a buttered rack. Poke with a fork, brush with the egg yolk, and spread with the black cumin seeds. Bake at 350°F (176°C) for 15 to 20 minutes.

BLACK CUMIN WREATH

1 pound (454 g) rye flour

1 teaspoon (5 g) salt

1 cup (240 ml) milk

3 tablespoons (45 g) butter

1 packet yeast

1 teaspoon (5 g) sugar

1 egg

$^1/_2$ pound (227 g) sourdough starter

1 egg yolk

2 tablespoons (30 g) black cumin seeds for sprinkling

Mix the ingredients into a dough and let it rise overnight, then knead it. Divide into 2 equal pieces, roll out, weave into a spiral pattern, and place like a wreath on the buttered rack. Let it rise again, brush with egg yolk, and sprinkle with black cumin seeds. Bake for 40 minutes at 350°F (176°C).

Exotic Spice

For soups, vegetable dishes, and stews, black cumin can be used instead of pepper. It is less spicy, but more easily digestible, which is important for people who suffer from stomach or kidney problems. Black cumin goes especially well with legumes and all types of cabbage. Its mild flavor makes it good in combinations with other spices such as savory, garlic, coriander, and thyme, and it is an essential component of curry and garam masala.

Meat Dishes

In the southeastern Mediterranean area it is customary to fry meat in olive oil and then add 2 teaspoons (30 ml) black cumin oil. Black cumin seeds also add an excellent flavor to patés and sausages.

Salads

Black cumin seeds add a hearty, unique taste to fresh salads. Add 1 tablespoon (15 g) black cumin seeds to the salad dressing. A splash of black cumin oil can refine salad dressings as well.

In the Canning Jar

Those who pickle their own vegetables can add a Middle Eastern touch by throwing in a sizable pinch of black cumin seeds. Because of its antibacterial effects black cumin also extends the storage life of foods.

Healthy Tea

Add boiling water to a mug with 1 tablespoon (15 g) black cumin seeds and let the tea sit for 10 minutes. The scent will transport you to the tents of the desert nomads, where healers to this day cure various ailments with black cumin.

Aromatic Coffee

In the bazaars and cafes of the Middle East, a pinch of black cumin powder is added to coffee according to individual preference. The desired amount of black cumin seeds can be added before grinding the coffee and black cumin together.

Resources

Pronatura Inc.
878 Sivert Drive
Wood Dale, IL 60191

Phone: (630) 766-3810
Fax: (630) 766-3850
Toll Free: (800) 555-7580
E-mail: pnatural@mindspring.com
www.pronaturainc.com

Supplier of black cumin products. Contact for availability in your area.